Baby Sleep Training

*What Works
(and what your grandparents
forgot to tell you)*

Table of Contents

Introduction 1

Chapter 1: Essential Overview of Sleep...2
   The Basics of Sleep 2
   Sleep's impact on Health...5
   Why Babies Cry 6
   An Infant's Sleep Space 8
   Sleep Safety and Co-sleeping 9
   Chapter One Summary 11

Chapter 2: Sleep In The First Three Months 13
   What To Expect For The First Three Months 13
   Night Sleeping For Babies Up To Three Months 15
   Naps In The First Three Months 18
   Sleeping Tips For Parents In The First Three Months. 20
   Summary: The First Three Months: 21

Chapter 3: Sleep In The 4th Through 6th Month 23
   The Power Of Consistency In Sleep Training 23
   Sleep In The 4th To 6th Month 24
   Sleep Training Overview 26
   Sample Sleep Training Week: CIO/Ferber 29
   Sample Sleep Training Week: No Tears 30
   Naps At 4 To 6 Months 31
   Summary: Fourth To Sixth Month 32

Chapter 4: Sleep in the 6th to 12th Month 33
   Sleep From 6 To 12 Months 33
   The 8th Month Sleep Regression 36
   Sleep Training For 10 To 12 Month Old Babies 37
   Summary: Sleep At 6 To 12 Months 37

Chapter 5: Sleep Training In Other Cultures And Common Baby Sleep Issues ..39
   Baby Sleep In Other Cultures..39
   Sleep Problems Common In Babies 42

Appendix: Sources Used 44
Conclusion 45

Introduction

Congratulations on buying *Baby Sleep Training* and thank you for doing so.

Getting your baby down for a good night's sleep or even a much needed nap can often be a lot harder than you might expect. Young babies just don't have the same internal clock older children and adults have to regulate sleep, and they can't yet tell us why they are having issues. This book will provide the answers and systematic instructions you can use to create your own sleep training method based on your baby.

Every baby is different and this book unlocks the secrets of effective sleep training, looking at several methods and written by a mom who had to struggle through sleep issues before. The tips and tricks in this book will improve the sleep of your infant as well as your own sleep.

There are plenty of books on this subject on the market, thanks again for choosing this one! Every effort was made to ensure it is full of as much useful information as possible, please enjoy!

Chapter 1: Essential Overview of Sleep

In order for the baby sleep training methods and strategies presented in the next chapters of this book to be most effective it is important to give a closer look to sleep itself, and not only as it relates to infants, but also adult sleep. Ideally, the point of this book is to give both the infant and their parents a good night's sleep. This chapter will briefly explore the whys and hows of sleep before focusing on infant's sleep including the importance sleep has for the infant's development, both physically and mentally as well as providing an overview of the best sleeping environment for infants and important safety concerns regarding the sleep of infants.

I do have to apologize for the denseness of at least the first part of this chapter. It is difficult to present the basics of sleep simply so this section will not be as easy to read as the rest of the book. Understanding sleep, however, will likely lead to better sleep for both you and your baby so it is well worth the slog.

The Basics of Sleep

Adults generally spend a third of their day sleeping, though most people do not give it much thought unless they are plagued by sleep issues. On a basic scientific level, sleep is a recurring state where both the mind and body reduce their interactions with the surrounding world. A sleeping person's voluntary muscles, which are the muscles consciously control and are generally the ones used in movement, cease most movements. The brain waves of a sleeping person show a great deal less activity than when they are awake. This period of less activity allows the body and brain to restore the wear and tear that accumulated during the day.

Sleep tends to happen in cycles with five stages. The first stage of sleep is light sleep. The sleeper is closest to wakefulness in this stage but the activities of the voluntary muscles slow from wakefulness though they will have an occasional twitch. This is the stage of the sleep cycle where the sleeper is most likely to wake because of an external stimulus such as a noise, light or even the need to pee. Thankfully, this is generally the shortest stage of the sleep cycle.

Sleep starts to deepen in the second stage. The sleeper's breathing and heart rate both slow and their body temperature lowers slightly as their body's metabolism slows down. The breathing and heart rate remain slow in the third stage when deep sleep is entered. Here, the brain waves exhibit a greater percentage of delta waves. Delta waves associate with the stage 3 deep sleep known as slow wave sleep. The fourth stage continues the slow wave sleep and the sleeper's voluntary muscles generally stop moving completely. In adults, these two stages are most common in the first couple of sleep cycles each night.

The final stage of sleep is known as rapid eye movement sleep or REM. REM sleep is when the sleeper dreams. Their brain activity increases with dreams while their heart rate and breathing both speed up. Muscles remain relaxed but exhibit more movement. Though the dreamer's eyes generally remain closed, REM sleep gets its name from the rapid movements of the eyes during the dreams. For adults, REM sleep is more common in the sleep cycles that happen in the later part of their night of sleep.

Each sleep cycle lasts about 90 minutes for adults, while sleep cycles for infants are generally 50 to 60 minutes in length. This is often one of the issues new parents have with they infant's sleep. If parents and infant fall asleep at the same time, the different length of the sleep cycle means that the infant will return to stage one about a half hour earlier than their parents. If there are noises or light present at that time or if the infant is in some sort of discomfort, a dirty diaper for example, they will wake and likely cry out, waking the parent from their deeper sleep which tends to be much more difficult than waking from REM or light sleep.

Another aspect of sleep that can be challenging for infants is the Circadian Rhythm. Almost all animals and plants, at least on the surface of the earth, have a set of metabolic responses in their body that are set to the position of the sun, sleep chiefly among them. Some animals are nocturnal and are active after the sun sets but inactive when it rises, while others are most active during dawn and dusk. These are called crepuscular. Most animals and plants, humans included, are diurnal or active primarily during the day. This is controlled by the Circadian rhythm.
About sleep in humans, the circadian rhythm is tied to the light/dark cycle of the sun. When the sun goes down, the hypothalamus sends a message to the brain to get ready to sleep. The brain then tells the body to start the production of melatonin, which helps to enable it to sleep. When the sun rises, the brain sends a signal to the body to decreases the production of melatonin, ceasing completely once the person has woken.

This is how it worked for thousands of generations, but in the last hundred and fifty years, humans have had more and more access to artificial light which can delay the production of melatonin by tricking the brain into thinking the sun hasn't set. Worse yet for sleep, in the last several years is the rise in the use of smart phones. Bright lights shining so close to the eyes before sleep, like the screen of a smart phone can further trick the mind into not readying the body for sleep. Those who have sleep issues might consider limiting phone use before bed or at least utilizing the night time dimming features on their phones before bed.

With infants, issues surrounding the circadian rhythm tend to happen in the first 6 to 8 months when the infant has not yet developed their own circadian rhythm. While they will develop one naturally, the circadian rhythm functions both as an ingrained as well as trained reaction. The difference is best shown with an example. A normal person's circadian rhythm provides a roughly 24-hour cycle. However, should that person go on a trip across several time zones, after a few days, their circadian rhythm will remain at a roughly 24-hour cycle, but will adapt to the natural light/dark cycle of their new time zone. An infant will develop a circadian rhythm as their body and mind develop and grow, but helping infants to develop the part of their own circadian rhythm that changes with their environment is one of the ultimate goals of sleep training.

Sleep's impact on Health

While a sleeping person's metabolism drops steeply compared to when they are awake, the body is not idle while they sleep. The body uses this time of little activity, to repair any damages that happened to the body when the person was awake. Strained muscles heal faster in sleep as do cuts or scrapes. In the brain, sleep gives the mind a chance to encode memories of things learned or experienced the previous day into the long-term memory. It also takes the time to ready the brain for its exertion the next day.

For children, and especially for infants, sleep aids greatly in their development and growth, both physically and mentally. As an infant sleeps, human growth hormones are coursing through their system enabling their rapid growth and feeding their eager minds. The great amount of growth and development early in life is one of the reasons babies sleep so much more than children and adults. The National Sleep foundation recommends that newborns get 17 hours of sleep a day, which reduces to 15 at 6 months, 14 at one year, and 13.5 at 18 months. Even above that age, they recommend that preschoolers get 10 to 13 hours and school age children get 9 to 10. Adults, on the other hand, are recommended to get 7 to 9 hours of sleep per night.

A note of caution to these sorts of recommendations: You likely noticed that the amounts for young children to adults come with a range. This is because no two people have the exact same need for sleep. Some people can function normally with 7 hours a night while others need a good 9 hours of sleep. While babies tend to sleep for much longer periods, their need for sleep will vary just as an adult's need for sleep.

Anyone who has gone without sleep for too long will likely be familiar with some of the effects lack of sleep has on people. It causes a lack of concentration and can have a negative impact on the memory, in both recalling things from the long-term memory, using the working memory, as well as encoding memories into the long-term memory. It can lead to mood changes, often leaving the person suffering from it to be irritable. The body tends to be less effected than the mind. This is because a lot of the internal repair of the body's cells that happen in sleep can also be accomplished during the day. Sleeplessness does have a major effect on the immune system though, making it work harder to perform the same functions. This can lead to the sleep-deprived person becoming more susceptible to getting sick.

For a baby's rapidly developing body and mind, the lack of sleep can be more serious. Studies have shown that sleep deprivation can have a negative impact on an infant's behavior, attention, memory, and ability to learn. Yet another reason, baby sleep training is so important.

Why Babies Cry

All new parents quickly become familiar with their baby's cry.

This relates to sleep because for young infants, crying is the only response they are capable of making and when there is an issue with their sleep, crying is how they will let you know that there is an issue. Understanding the possible reasons for their crying will allow you to fix the problem and enable your baby, as well as yourself, to get back to sleep quicker.

Generally speaking, babies cry when they are experiencing some sort of discomfort. This could be because of hunger, a messy diaper, or an injury or illness. Other less tangible discomforts may also cause a baby to cry.

Babies often desire contact, to be held, to be near their parents. While it might be hard to imagine yourself as an infant, the best way to understand their need to be held would be to do so. Imagine being an infant and experiencing the world anew while being in a body that you can hardly control. They are so dependent on their parents that sometimes they need to know that their parents are their, that they are safe.

Overstimulation is a similar cause of crying, though less so for crying while they are supposed to be sleeping. Try again to think about seeing the world as an infant. With so many new stimuli, becoming overwhelmed is an understandable problem. Moving the infant to a quieter place for a few minutes can do wonders to help in situations where an infant is overstimulated.

To help alleviate crying related to hunger, learning some of the signs of hunger, prior to crying can be helpful. A hungry baby is often fussy. There is also a reflexive reaction called rooting, if your baby turns their head towards your hand when you stroke their cheek, they are often hungry.

Somewhat related to hunger, post-feeding gas can also be an issue that causes discomfort in infants. Babies breast to bottle fed swallow a lot of air, burping after feeding will help as will laying them on their back and moving their legs in a bicycling motion.

If no cause to the crying can be found, it is possible that the infant has a scratch or is being irritated by a tag on their clothes. Check their toes and fingers for hairs or threads that might have wrapped around them. These hair tourniquets can cut off circulation and cause the infant pain, but if the baby is wearing socks, it isn't an issue.

For babies in the 4 to 7-month stage, the start of teething can lead to crying, so touching your baby's gums to feel them might give you an idea of why they are crying if no other cause can be found.

An Infant's Sleep Space

One of the best ways to ensure that your infant will be sleeping like a champ is to ensure that their sleep space is as conducive as possible for a good night sleep. There are three basic aspects of this: temperature, darkness, and silence. All of these come down to minimizing the external stimuli that can cause an infant to wake up during the night and—as they have not developed any other way to express their discomfort—crying out to their parents.

The ideal temperature for sleep is between 68–72 degrees Fahrenheit (20–22 degrees Celsius). Remember that the body temperature drops slightly during sleep, so over heating the infant can lead to sleep problems among other issues that will be discussed in the next section. As for blankets, infants tend to gain the ability to grasp blankets and recover themselves between the age of 2 and 4 so for younger infants a sleep sack or other sleep clothing is preferred over blankets. When a baby kicks off their blanket and gets too cold, they will wake and cry out. With a sleep sack, the baby's blanket can't be kicked off, so they won't get too cold and wake you with their cries.

Darkness is sleeps best friend. As discussed above in the section about the circadian rhythm, darkness stimulates sleep by the brain instructing the body to produce melatonin, which aids in sleep. Even for infants whose circadian rhythm has not developed fully, darkness minimizes the possible external stimuli that can wake a baby during the light sleeping segment of the sleep cycle.

Noises are one of the main things that can wake adults up from their sleep and babies have much more sensitive hearing than adults do. Minimizing the external sounds can lead to better sleep for your baby. Sometimes it is impossible to do this. If you live in an apartment near a busy city street, the night noises of the city will be a constant background noise to your nights. A white noise machine or fan can be a solution here; the gentle constant droning noise will mask external sounds enabling the baby to sleep through those noises. Music might work for older children and adults, but it is generally too distracting for infants.

Sleep Safety and Co-sleeping

Sudden Infant Death Syndrome (SIDS) is thankfully a rare problem that only results in 90 deaths a year per 100,000 live births in the United States. This number has gone down dramatically in the last 20 years as scientists have begun to understand more and more of the risk factors. The following guidelines take into account the most recent information and thinking about SIDS and provide a way to minimize this already small, yet terrifying risk.

Many parents find co-sleeping, bringing their infant into their bed to sleep, to be beneficial and there are certainly pros. There are some cons as well, including in certain circumstances an increased chance of SIDS. These pros and cons will be explored after the SIDS prevention recommendations.

The biggest decline in SIDS deaths came from a better understanding of sleep position. Infants under a year old should sleep on a firm mattress, and should be placed on their back. As they age, they will be better able to move during the night. Once your baby can roll over in their sleep, there is generally not an issue with how they sleep, but should still be placed on their back in their crib.

Do not use any foam wedges or rolled up towels to prevent your baby's movement in their crib as these have been found to increase the risk of SIDS. Removing all soft toys from the crib as the infant sleeps is also recommended.

Overheating can lead to an increased SIDS risk, so using a sleep sack can minimize the risk. Some studies have found that immunizations also minimize the risk, so keep up on those vaccinations.

A fan, either box or ceiling, contributes to air circulation and has been found to reduce risk of SIDS.

Breast-feeding is beneficial and while the reasons for that are unknown, it is theorized that breast-feeding helps the baby fight infections that might lead to an increased risk of SIDS. If you are breast-feeding, avoiding alcohol keeps the SIDS risk low.

Cigarette smoke is detrimental to infant's health in several ways and has been found to increase SIDS risk. Not to preach, but it is bad for adults as well, but at the very least keep it away from babies.

When it comes comes to co-sleeping, should you choose to do

this, following all of the above SIDS safety guidelines is the best practice. In addition, co-sleeping should not be done with infants under 6 months or those born underweight or premature. It is also not recommended for smokers, as an increased risk of SIDS has been found among co-sleeping babies if one of the parents is a smoker, even if they do not smoke around the baby or even in the house.

The consumption of alcohol prior to sleeping in the same bed with an infant is also discouraged as is taking any medication that causes drowsiness or sleep. These factors contribute to smothering deaths.

One last con for co-sleeping is that it can have negative effects on the sex life of the parents. Babies tend to be intuitive of the emotions of others and especially their parents. Any increased stress in their parent's relationship can be internalized by the baby and contribute to sleep issues.

The last couple of paragraphs paint a scary picture of co-sleeping, but there are benefits. Bringing an infant into the bed leads to a closer connection to the child so early in their life. The infant being near will also enable the parent to respond to their needs quicker, leading to easier feedings and less time for the baby to cry and wake themselves further. Babies have a desire for touch and the closeness co-sleeping provides can satisfy this need leading to better sleep. Finally, some studies have found that sleeping in the same room as their parents lowers the risk of SIDS. Even if you do not intend to co-sleep, keeping your baby's crib in the room you sleep in for the first year can provide many of the benefits of co-sleep without many of the cons.

Chapter One Summary

- Sleep occurs in cycles, 90 minutes for adults and between

50 and 60 minutes for babies, with a short period of light sleep occurring in each cycle. This short period is when babies tend to wake and cry.

- Sleep is governed by the circadian rhythm that keeps an internal clock tied to the sun's light/dark cycle. Darkness causes the body to release melatonin to ready it for sleep. The circadian rhythm usually develops in about the sixth month of life, so newborns will not respond to it.
- Generally, the best sleeping environment for an infant is at room temperature (68-72 degrees Fahrenheit), in a room with little light and either no external noise or white noise used to mask external noises.
- Co-sleeping can be beneficial as it keeps your baby close and allows you to feed and help them during the night as well as lead to greater connection to your baby.
- Do not co-sleep after consuming alcohol, taking medication that causes drowsiness, or if you or your partner is a smoker. Do not co-sleep with a baby on a couch or in an armchair and never leave a baby on a bed unsupervised.
- SIDS prevention tips: Babies under one year in age should be placed to sleep on their back on top of a firm mattress though when they can roll over under their own power, moving them back to sleeping on their back is unnecessary. Do not leave any soft toys or use wedges or towels to keep the baby in place while in the crib. Use a fan, box, or ceiling, to circulate air in the baby's room. Do not smoke around the baby. Breastfeeding is beneficial in reducing the risk of SIDS

Chapter 2: Sleep In The First Three Months

All right, time to move on from the basics of sleep and get into infant sleep training. This chapter will deal with what to expect from your baby's sleep in the first three months of their life. This touches on general sleep habits of infants of that age as well as a look at both day and night sleep along with tips on starting effective sleeping habits as your baby reaches 6 to 8 weeks old. There is even a short section of tips for parents to maximize their own sleep.

What To Expect For The First Three Months

Hands down, when it comes to your baby's sleep habits, the first three months will likely be the most chaotic. An old adage states, "All babies are born three months too early," and there is a lot of truth to that. When human babies are born, they can't walk or even crawl and usually takes several months before they can even roll themselves over.

Comparing this to some other mammals shows a stark difference. Newborn elephants and horses, for example, can walk within minutes of being born. Predators, such as cats and bears are often born as helpless as human babies are—not able to walk or even open their eyes. However, that situation changes fast. Only in the great apes, humanity's closest cousins, are there species that have such helpless babies. Chimpanzee mothers carry their babies everywhere they go for the first year of their life and even then, chimp babies rarely venture more than 20 feet away from their mother for the first three years of their lives.

The reason human and ape babies are so dependent on others is that they are not done developing and staying in the womb would cause many problems when it came to birth. If you have a three-month old baby, imagine giving birth to them today instead of three months ago. Most babies double in weight during that time! There are also benefits for the baby to continue with their development outside the womb. Babies, even before they are born, are always learning. They listen to their surroundings and when they can, they watch, touch, and lick them too. Their interactions with other early in their life, especially with their parents, shape and mold their understanding of the world and most of that couldn't happen in the womb.

In regard to sleep, during their first three months of life babies tend to sleep most of the time but unlike older babies, children and adults, as they are still in a major development phase, there is little pattern to their sleep. Babies in this age bracket have not established a circadian rhythm and have no sleep habits to cue themselves to start one. Attempting to create sleep habits is the goal of sleep training in this stage of a baby's life though it is only at the 6 to 8-week mark that these habits can be made, before that point, baby sleep training is limited to trying to get them to sleep then back to sleep when they wake up crying.

In the first two weeks of life, a baby will generally sleep between 16 to 18 hours a day. The only real pattern to sleep at this age is their feeding schedule. Newborn babies have tiny stomachs, which combined with their usual voracious appetite generally means they need to be fed every three hours or so, regardless of the time. After about two weeks, most babies will start to form what will become a sleep pattern. At this age, they will tend to sleep about 9 hours a night and roughly 6 to 7 hours in the day split between three or four daily naps. AS the baby approaches three months old, their nightly amount of sleep stabilizes at between 8-10 hours and their daytime naps reduce in length and amount with generally two to three naps totally 5 hours.

Baby Sleep Training

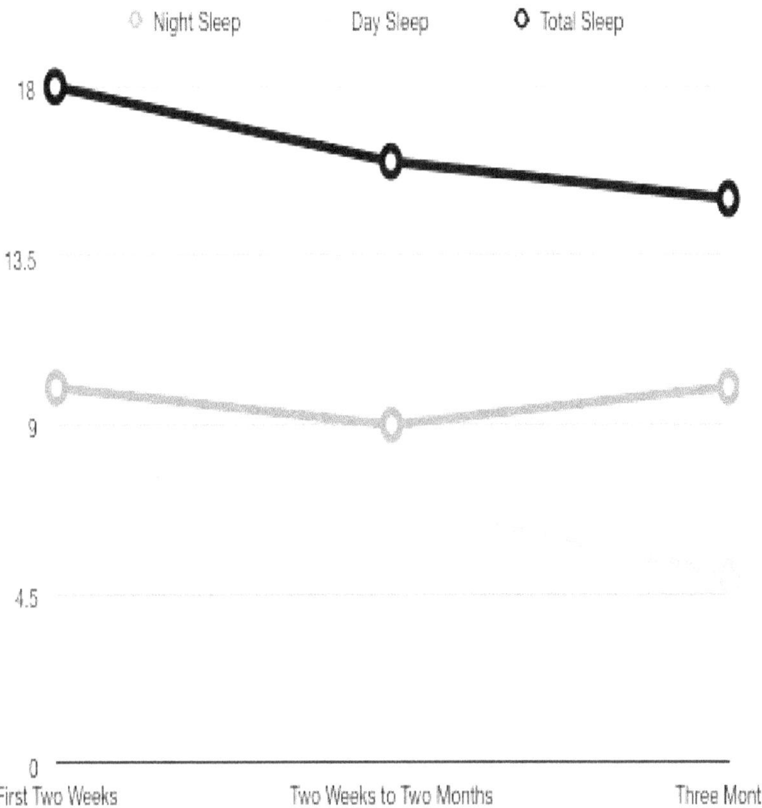

Please note, and this is something that is likely going to be repeated over and over again, just as adult sleep patterns differ, no baby has the exact same type of sleep pattern as other babies. Comparing your baby's sleep habits with other's children, and especially fretting about the differences, does little good. The exception here is where there are drastic differences, for instance if your three month old barely sleeps at all, in which case, taking your baby to the pediatrician is the best option.

Night Sleeping For Babies Up To Three Months

While starting the actual sleep training will have to wait until they are a few months old, the best way to ensure good habits even this early in their lives is to establish a strong sleep routine. This includes providing the baby with a nighttime environment that is as conducive to sleep as possible. A lot of the tips and suggestions in this chapter apply to the entire age range while some are more suitable for either the first few weeks to a month and others are of more use after 6 to 8 weeks when your baby has developed enough to start forming habits. Any of the tips or suggestions that focused on a more specific age range will be mentioned.

Providing an environment conducive for sleep is not that difficult. Most babies of almost any age sleep best in a room that is about average room temperature (68–72 degrees Fahrenheit or 20–22 degrees Celsius) and is dark and quiet. Often, the most difficult of these to provide is silence. We often live in a loud world, even in the middle of the night. If external noises are an issue in your home, a white noise machine, or even a box fan, might be the solution for your baby sleeping woes. Quiet white or fan noise can mask external sounds so your baby's sleep isn't interrupted by the sounds of the early morning street sweeper outside their window. And of course, following all of the recommendations to minimize the risk of SIDS discussed in the first chapter

For babies under 60 days old, swaddling them before bed can help them sleep better and for longer. People, including babies, are creatures of habit and while adults tend to have forgotten their time as infants, a newborn baby remembers being in the womb and often takes comfort in the constricting feel of the swaddle. A swaddle that constricts the use of the arms is only recommended for the first 60 days as continuing it afterwards can have negative effects on the baby's motor development.

Here are the instructions for a simple diamond swaddle:

- Set your baby's blanket on a flat surface. A square blanket is preferred but you can fold a rectangular blanket into a square.
- Arrange the blanket into a diamond shape with one of the corners pointing towards you.
- Flip the top corner down towards you about 5 or 6 inches.
- Place your baby on the blanket with their head above the flipped down corner.
- Pull the right corner of the blanket over your baby and tuck it under your baby's left side.
- Grab the bottom corner and pull it over the baby's left shoulder.
- Finally take the left corner and pull it across your baby's body then lift your baby and tuck it underneath them.

Make sure not to try to straighten your baby's legs in a swaddle as this can damage their joints and even cause hip dysplasia. This is an abnormality in the baby's hip joint, which results in an increased risk of joint dislocation.

During the first few weeks, feel free to try almost anything to get your baby to sleep. Rock them, sing to them, rub their back, put them in their car seat on top of the dryer, anything to get through the night. After the first few weeks though, it is best to start to curtail these methods. As your baby ages, these tricks can form habits where your baby will come to expect those actions before they fall asleep making it difficult for them to go to sleep and more importantly for you, go back to sleep, without you rocking them or whatever sleep crutch they have begun to inspect.

Shushing during the first few weeks can work wonders in calming your baby. This is likely because the shushing sound is similar to the sounds your baby heard in the womb. A baby's ears develop early in the third trimester and the sound of their mother's blood circulating through her body is believed to be as loud as a vacuum cleaner to their new ears. Like swaddling, the shushing sound reminds them of their time in the womb.

After the first month, it can be beneficial to try to set them down to sleep at least once a day when they are drowsy but still awake. This can be more difficult than it sounds as sometimes your baby will be fussy and might even cry a little but it will start to allow them to learn to fall asleep on their own, which will help a lot later on. Learn your baby's sleep signals. Some of the most common are eye rubbing, fussiness and of course yawning. Putting them down to bed when they start to show these signals will help to establish a sleep routine.

At 6 to 8 weeks, most babies' sleep habits start to become more predictable. Try to put your baby to sleep at night when they are still awake but are showing signs of drowsiness. This is the age when a bedtime routine becomes vital and will help to give your baby strong sleep habits. The routine will differ, baby to baby, but it is best that it be calming in general. A common bedtime routine starts with a bath, then a feeding and finally reading your baby a story. Performing a bedtime routine with your baby will get them into the habit of getting themselves ready to sleep. As the habit is repeated, it becomes stronger and when they develop their own circadian rhythm, a preexisting habit will only make that quicker and easier.

Naps In The First Three Months

Again, in the first couple of weeks, while your baby will spend most of their time sleeping, there will be little pattern to when they sleep. At this early stage, it is best to let them sleep. That is when their little bodies and minds grow the most in the first few weeks. Don't worry about sticking to a feeding schedule in these first weeks, letting them sleep a little longer is better than waking them. The same is true for wet diapers, today's diapers are quite good at avoiding moisture, and there is no harm in letting your baby sleep a little longer and changing them then.

Here, again, it must be stressed that all babies are different. Some take fewer but longer naps and others take several shorter naps, there is no problem with that sort of variation, only when your baby is either barely sleeping or always sleeping are there likely problems and a pediatrician should be consulted.

After the anarchic first few weeks, most babies sleep pattern slowly becomes predictable and their naps tend to consolidate by the 6th to 8th week. At this point, a nap schedule can be established. Watching for your baby's signals of drowsiness such as eye rubbing and yawning, maybe they always fall asleep during a car trip at a specific time. It is easier to establish a nap schedule that conforms to the times that they are most tired during the day.

As part of this nap schedule, a simpler version of the bedtime routine can help to reinforce it as putting them down for a nap in the same space that they sleep at night. Feeding them and then telling a story before setting them in their crib is a common abbreviated bedtime ritual for naptime.

If your baby is in day care, and that day care includes a naptime, putting them down at the same time on the days they are not in day care will help to keep them on a nap schedule. Consistency is key, though an occasional disruption to their schedule does little harm as long is it truly is occasional.

If your baby is being particularly fussy, a pacifier can help to soothe them as babies find the act of sucking calming. Be cautious with its use as a crutch, however. Other ways to soothe a fussy baby to get them ready to sleep include infant swings and putting them on their side or stomach. Both of these shouldn't be used for sleep, only for soothing. Like many tricks with young babies, these harken back to the womb and are calming to most babies.

Sleeping Tips For Parents In The First Three Months.

Establishing a good sleep schedule for your baby benefits them greatly, but it might benefit you even more. You don't require nearly as much sleep as your baby, but their inclusion into your life is a huge disruption to the sleep schedule you have likely been following since early adulthood. Here are some tips to catch your z's in your baby's first three months.

One of the easier ways to get enough sleep in the first three months, and especially in the first couple of weeks, is to try to catch a nap when your baby does. Set up a baby monitor, or sleep in the same room as your baby. If they wake up and start to cry, it will wake you and you can handle their needs. No harm will come to your baby by crying for a few minutes while you wake.

Just as the best sleep environment for your baby is a dark and quiet, coolish room, the same can be said for most adults. Following the same guidelines for your own rest will likely improve its quality even when your baby is making sure that you don't get the quantity of sleep you desire. For nighttime sleep, limiting your use of bright lights a few hours before bedtime will aid your circadian rhythm in producing melatonin. Use your phone or computer's nighttime settings when using them after dark. These settings dim the screen and shift the colors to a warmer spectrum. Like shutting off bright lights, this will aid in the production of melatonin.

Accepting the help of others and limiting your responsibilities in the first month or so can also help your sleep. Trading off responsibilities with your partner can help both of your sleep habits. For example, if you are breast-feeding, pump your milk before going to sleep and let your partner handle the next feeding while you sleep. If you or your partner is a light sleeper, an occasional night in a separate room from both partner and baby can be used to sleep off some of the sleep deficit you have accrued.

When it comes to responsibilities, a lot of new mothers try and jump right back into regular life after giving birth and the stress involved in trying that as well as caring for a new baby can easily lead to sleep issues. Parents of their second child might feel as if they are neglecting their oldest and try to schedule activities with them so they are not left out. Taking a few weeks to a month to acclimate to the new child is perfectly acceptable and less extra responsibilities will help you get sleep when you can manage it.

Summary: The First Three Months:

- In the first couple of weeks your baby will sleep most of the time, but with little pattern except for their hunger.
- After two weeks they will sleep an average of 15-18 hours with about 9 at night and the rest in three or four naps during the day
- At three months, their sleeping becomes more predictable, sleeping about 10 hours at night and 5 hours during the day in two or three naps.
- Remember, all babies are different and some will sleep longer or shorter than others will. This is fine.
- Don't worry about bad habits in the first couple of weeks. Just get them to sleep.
- Dark and quite rooms at a comfortably cool temperature are best to promote longer and better quality sleep
- Start a bedtime and shorter naptime ritual after the first

month or so to get your baby into the habit of sleeping on a schedule.

- Consistency builds habits. Try to keep nap and bed time at the same time each day.
- Avoid sleep crutches after the first month and put your baby to bed drowsy, yet still awake, so they learn to fall asleep on their own.
- Try and catch a nap when your baby naps
- Trade off responsibilities with your partner to help both of you get more sleep
- If you can, minimize outside responsibilities in the first month, taking on too much too early will cost you in sleep.

Chapter 3: Sleep In The 4ᵗʰ Through 6ᵗʰ Month

In the forth to the sixth month most babies sleep patterns start become less chaotic and they have reached the age where sleep training can start in earnest. This chapter will touch on what to expect from your 4 to 6-month old baby, provided an overview on a few of the most common sleep training methods and then two step by step examples using different combinations of methods.

Again, all babies are different and progress at different rates. Some might be able to handle sleep training as early as 4 months while others might need until the 6th or 7th month. The best method of sleep training will vary as well. Some babies respond better to certain systems. Instead of focusing all your efforts on pursuing one sleep training method over another, a combination of different methods is often the best.

The Power Of Consistency In Sleep Training

People tend to be creatures of habit and this starts almost at birth. For babies, almost everything is a new experience and the world seems to be a chaotic place. This can cause a lot of stress, which can have negative effects on their emotions, which can lead to sleep problems. Providing babies with a routine, a general daily schedule, can insulate then from this stress and keep them happier.

When it comes to sleep, a consistent routine where you put the baby down to sleep, at night and for naps, at about the same time every day. With babies whose circadian rhythm hasn't fully developed yet, this can have the added benefit of aiding in its development. For babies whose circadian rhythm has started, keeping a consistent schedule of sleep and nap times will help to reinforce their nascent circadian rhythm.

As stated many times, all babies are different so when formulating a sleep schedule, it can be much easier for all involved if you approach the routine less as a schedule you will dictate to your baby and more of a collaborative project. Some babies will naturally take fewer, longer naps while others might take more, shorter naps. Trying to force your baby's nap habits into a schedule that is not natural for them will likely result in an increase in both your and your baby's stress level and cost you both some sleep.

As your baby's natural sleep schedule starts to become more predictable in these months, watch it somewhat closely, and take a few notes over a couple of days. Try to discover your baby's signs of tiredness so you can put them down to sleep before they get too tired and become cranky.

Another thing to look for is changes in your baby's sleep habits. Even after they stabilize, they can change. You baby might have been set in a pattern of three 60-minute-naps each day but start to sleep longer in their earlier 2 maps and just won't fall asleep when you put them down for their third nap. Don't force their previous schedule for the sake of consistency, adapt.

Sleep In The 4th To 6th Month

There are several welcome changes to your baby's sleep habits that generally occur in the 4th to 6th months. At this point, their circadian rhythm is starting to develop and their stomachs tend to have grown. Both of these changes lead to your baby sleeping for longer and longer times overnight. Most babies at 4 months can sleep about 8 hours without interruption, while most 6-

month olds can sleep for 10 hours without interruptions for parents. This can give the parents much better sleep because of fewer interruptions from a crying baby.

One change that will likely have a negative effect on your baby's sleep is teething. Most babies' teeth start coming in between 4 to 6 months and this can cause them a lot of discomfort and pain. Some have found white noise generators helpful in distracting their babies from their gum pain as they fall asleep.

Maintaining a consistent bedtime and nap schedule will work to reinforce these development changes. Keeping a bedtime ritual aids this further. By now, this should be a habit for your baby and just starting the ritual will begin to trigger their drowsiness. Again, all babies are different and you should consider this as you work on your baby's bedtime ritual. The common one, bath, feeding, and then a story, might work great with your baby but on the other hand, a bath might make them a bit hyperactive. If reading a story as part of the ritual, remember that your goal is to help your baby wind down and relax. Telling an exciting story that uses loud sound effects is counterproductive to getting them to sleep. Pay attention to how your bedtime ritual effects your baby and modify it accordingly.

When it comes to your baby's sleeping environment, there is no change from the suggestions for the earlier months. A cool, quiet and dark room is the most conducive to sleep. A fan or white noise machine can be helpful in masking external noises that can't be helped as well as the occasional unavoidable noises. It is best to set your baby to sleep on their back but usually around this age is when you baby will have the ability to roll over. Don't worry about pushing them back onto their back to sleep if they do roll over.

One way to assist your baby in sleeping through the night at this age is to cluster feed in the afternoon and early evening. Babies at this age have a larger stomach so can be fed more in one sitting. Adding a couple of feedings in the evening will fill their stomach enough that they won't wake up hungry in the middle of the night.

In general, 4-month-old babies will sleep about 15 hours a day with 9 to 10 at night and the rest in several short naps. As they reach 6 months, the total hours will drop slightly, to 13 or 14 hours a day. Again, 9 to 10 of these will happen at night while the rest will be naps. The amount of daily naps tends to go down by 6 months and stabilize at two or three. Of course, all babies are different, so their sleeping patterns will vary.

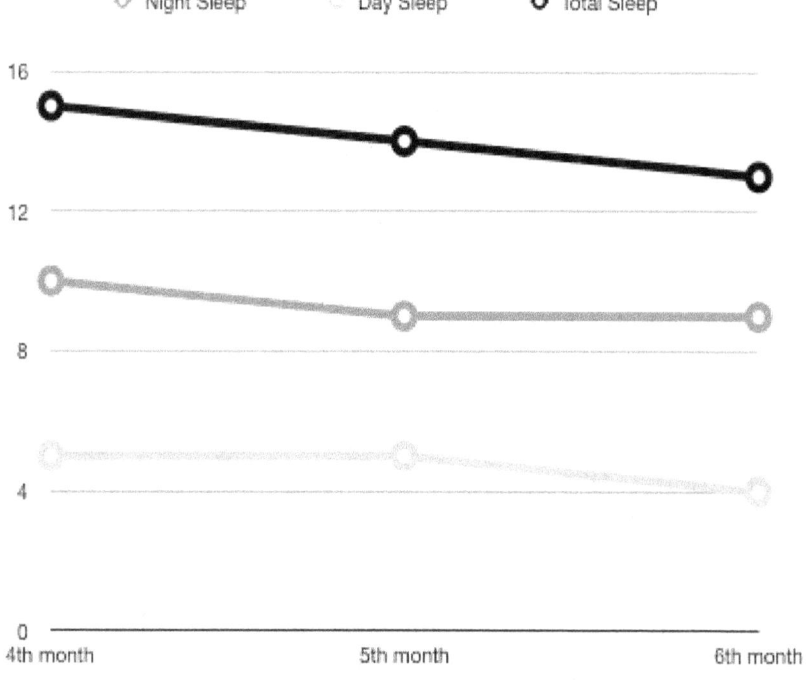

Sleep Training Overview

There are competing schools of thought when it comes to sleep training. While there are several different methods, the disagreement tends to focus on crying. Some methods favor a system where the parents ignore their baby's cry after being put down at night while others favor a tear free, gentler, method that weans the baby off of rely on their parent to get them to sleep.

The end goal for both types of systems is the same: self-soothing. Sleep training teaches the baby to not rely on their parents when falling asleep. Once a baby can self-sooth, they are much less likely to cry out when they wake up in the middle of the night, instead they will fall back asleep. A further benefit of this is that the baby that can self sooth will also rely less on any sleeping crutches and will usually be much easier to put down to bed every night.

For the no tears methods, the general idea is to slowly wean your baby off any sleep crutches that they have developed. These can vary by baby, some like to be gently swung before they fall asleep, shushing helps with others. For the sake of example, rocking will be used here. In the last chapter, putting your baby down to sleep while they were awake, yet drowsy, was discussed as a way to introduce your baby to self-soothing. This is continued in the no tears methods, as is the introduction of a bedtime ritual.

As the no tears method begins, the parent starts to use their baby's sleep crutch less and less until they cease using it completely. Using rocking as an example at the store of the no tears sleep training, rock them for the same amount you normally do, then put them away. Repeat the rocking if they wake in the night and need to be put back to bed. As the training progresses, rock them less each time before returning them to their crib or rock them at a slower pace. Make sure to keep putting them to sleep when they are still awake, even though this is the no tears method, self-soothing is still the end goal. Another no cry method advocates camping out next to the crib as you put your baby to sleep so that they know you are there. As sleep training progresses each night, you move further and further away from the crib until you are no longer in the room. If your baby cries out into the night, comfort them as you normally would or combine with the other no cry method and comfort them in shorter and shorter intervals.

The cry it out methods, on the other hand, require the parent to ignore their baby's crying. Some of these methods, like the Weissbluth method, involve ignoring their cries for the entire night but most, like the Ferber method, advocate leaving your baby alone in their room after you put them down to sleep and leaving for an interval. Initially let your baby cry for five minutes, before entering and comforting them. The next day, wait 10 minutes to come and comfort them.

There are many benefits to the cry it out method as well as a few downsides. It generally works quickly, often in less than a week. This leads to better sleep in both quality and quantity which aid in baby development. It also gets rid of sleep crutches and bad habits before they become routine. Better baby sleep usually goes together with better sleep for their parents, too.

On the negative, listening to your baby cry is often quite difficult. There is also the issue of your baby's distress and stress level. There is a lot of disagreement here among experts and scientists as to the possible negative effects of prolonged crying. Some see little to no long term negative effects from it while others worry that the cortisol, a stress hormone, released during prolong crying can have negative effects on a baby's mental development as well as their emotional health.

One of the ways to minimize this possibility is to learn to

differentiate your baby's cries. If you can tell the difference between their cry for attention and their cry for discomfort, you can let them cry it out when they just want attention and go to them if they are crying out of distress. The generally short intervals used in the Ferber method will likely not have negative effects and since the "cry it out" methods generally work quickly. The crying will only be for a couple of nights.

Again, every baby is different so they might not react to the method you try. In the end, mixing methods will often provide the best solution to your baby's sleep training. Comparing your baby's progress to other babies is never a good idea. There is nothing wrong with your baby if they do not have a sleep schedule at 5 months just because your cousin's baby had one at 4 months.

Sample Sleep Training Week: CIO/Ferber

Before starting your week of cry it out baby sleep training, establish your baby's sleep routines. Get into the habit of providing a nightly bedtime ritual as well as an abbreviated naptime ritual to get your baby into a relaxed state. As part of this, start putting your baby down to sleep when they are still awake but drowsy.

On the first day of training, go through your bedtime ritual and put your baby down to sleep, then leave the room. If your baby starts to cry, wait 5 minutes before reentering the room. Comfort your baby verbally and with touch, but do not pick them up and then put them back down to bed. If they continue to cry, again, wait five minutes before entering the room and comforting them, again do not pick them up.

Day 2 follows the same pattern except you wait 10 minutes before coming in to comfort your baby. This interval extends by 5 minutes a day until it reaches 30 minutes. If at that point, your baby hasn't started to learn to self-sooth, modifying the method is likely the best option. The cry it out method doesn't always work, no method is fool proof

Sample Sleep Training Week: No Tears

Just as with the cry it out method the no tears method works best when your baby has an established sleep routine including a nightly bed time ritual and putting your baby down to sleep while they are still awake but drowsy. This method tends to take longer than the cry it out methods so be prepared to keep going at it for longer. For the sample week, this will include both camping out and fading.

On day one, after you complete your baby's bedtime ritual, put them down to sleep as you normally would and sit in a chair right next to their crib. If they fall asleep without crying, great, go about your evening as you normally would. If they cry out in the night, go to them and offer comfort as you normally would in the way that normally gets them back to sleep.

Day 2, again, bedtime routine and sleepy but awake when you put them in their crib. Move the chair a couple of feet away from the crib. If your baby cries, comfort them as you normally would but incrementally less. If you normally rock them for 5 minutes, cut 30 seconds from that and rock them with slightly less motion. Put them back into the crib and sit back down. One they are asleep, leave the room. If they cry at night, offer the same, incrementally less, comfort.

Each day after this, move the chair further back from the crib and offer smaller and smaller amount of comfort each day. Ideally, at some point, your baby will start to self-sooth and won't cry when put down in their crib. As your chair gets further and further away, you will end up out of the room. At that point, just leave the room after putting your baby down to sleep.

Naps At 4 To 6 Months

Naps tend to lengthen in these months, as shorter naps just don't work for babies in this stage of developments. Most babies move to two or three naps per day of about 90 minutes in length. Of course, all babies are different so some might nap longer or shorter. This is fine. As your baby's nap schedule changes, look for the signs of tiredness and use them to modify their nap schedule accordingly.

Summary: Fourth To Sixth Month

- Most Babies sleep patterns become more consistent between the fourth and sixth months.
- At 4 months, most babies sleep about 15 hours a day with 9-10 of them at night and the rest in several daytime naps.
- By 6 months, most babies sleep around 13 hours a day, 9-10 at night and the rest in 2 to 3 longer naps during the daytime.
- Sleep training is possible for most babies at this time
- Cry it out sleep training allows your baby to learn to self sooth at night by leaving them on their own after putting to bed for short intervals that increase each day.

No tears sleep training offers a gentler approach where you still comfort your baby, but incrementally offer less and less of your baby's sleep crutch as you continue the training.

Chapter 4: Sleep in the 6th to 12th Month

After 6 months, your baby is likely inching towards toddlerhood. While they still have a long way to go, some major parts of their mental and physical development has already happened. They will be much more mobile and vocal in the latter half of their first year as their independence starts to show itself.

Sleep From 6 To 12 Months

Most 6-month-old babies tend to sleep about 13-14 hours a day total with 9-10 at night and the rest in 2 to 3 naps during the day. By the time they reach their first birthday the total will likely have fallen to 12 hours total with 9 hours at night and the rest in a couple of daytime naps.

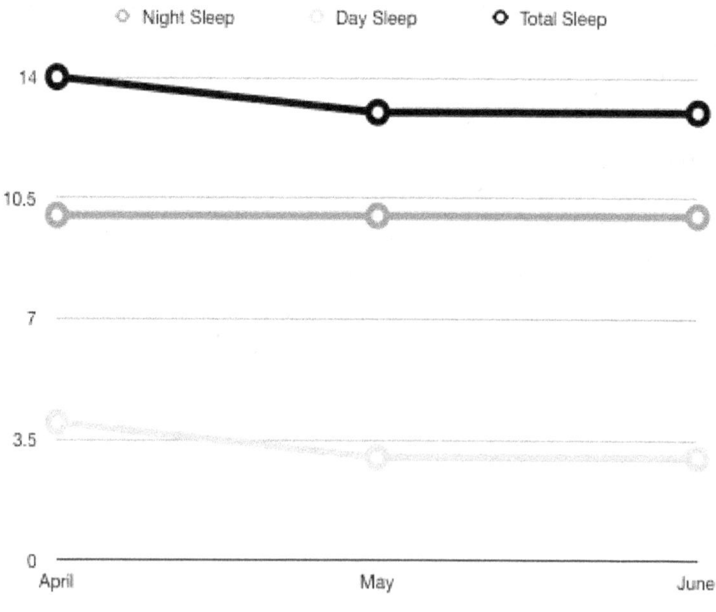

Babies at this age are beginning to become mobile, learning to crawl and explore their world. They will likely move more around the crib. With this greater mobility, it is safer to allow stuffed toys in the crib at night. For those who prefer a no tears sleep training method, adding a special stuffed toy or blanket can aid in this, giving your baby something to focus on to get comfort instead of relying on their parents.

Consistency remains key in continuing proper sleep habits. Maintaining the same bed times, including the bedtime ritual to calm your baby before bed, is central to this. As you baby develops, their nap schedule will change. Most babies between 6 to 12 months old will likely take 2 to 3 naps during the day but expect changes to this. Modifying their nap schedule as they develop will keep fussiness to a minimum.

Continuing to watch and understand your baby's sleep signs will help to modify their nap schedule. Each baby is different and might have different sleep signs but some of the most common at this age are pulling at ears, fluttering eyelids, boredom with toys, fussiness and of course yawning. If your baby starts showing these signs well before their scheduled nap for a few days in a row, it might be a good idea to switch to an earlier naptime. Similarly, if your baby is too alert and wired at the time of their scheduled nap for a couple of days in a row, shifting it back an hour might help.

One of the side effects of your baby's growing independence is that they will start to show and assert their preferences. This can create disruptions and changes to their bedtime ritual as well as their nighttime sleep environment. While consistency is still key, making small modifications to the bedtime ritual or your baby's sleeping environment can be helpful if the previous one is no longer calming your baby.

Babies at this age can generally sleep for 7 to 8 hours

uninterrupted and will only need one nighttime feeding though an occasional extra is possible. As they age closer to a year, they will likely be ready to be night weaned. Babies ready for night weaning often start to eat less during the day and when they wake at night for feeding, they will treat it more as playtime. Getting them to eat more during the day, using cluster feedings in the afternoon and evening will help. Their waking at night can be out of habit. Increasing the amount, they eat in the afternoon will keep them full enough to not wake in hunger at night.

If you are having consistent issues at bet time with your 6 to 9-month old baby that just can't settle down, try to put them to bed a half hour earlier, continuing with your bedtime ritual, just a little earlier. Their inability to sleep might be a sign of them being over tired.

The 8th Month Sleep Regression

Sleep regression is a common problem that parents face in the 8th to 9th month of their baby's life. This is a period when they might experience more wakefulness at night along with shorter, or even skipped, naps. Thankfully, this short-term issue generally lasts between 2 to 6 weeks so it is likely to pass.

The cause for sleep regression is the baby's development. Their bodies and brains have undergone so many growths and changes in their short life but around the 8th month, they will generally start to better explore their world. Their muscles are now strong enough for them to crawl, allowing them to move on their own power. Their brains have been absorbing language since their ears developed in the womb, but they have now developed to the point where they can start to speak words. All these changes and new experiences often leave their minds a bit too wired to calm down and fall asleep.

Patience is often the only remedy to deal with this sleep regression. It will pass on its own. To minimize it, continue with your bedtime rituals, consistency is still key, but be open to modify them slightly. At this age, your baby will be starting to assert their independence. Certain parts of your bedtime routine might not work as they had before given your baby's changing tastes. When it comes to naps, the sleep regression is often a point when your baby's nap schedule changes permanently. Shifting to a new nap schedule is a possibility.

When it comes to the different sleep training methods, the sleep regression can be a large disruption to them. If your previous sleep training had been more of a no tears method, the sleep regression is likely not a good time to try a cry it our method. This is a temporary situation and regular sleep will likely return once it is over. Should that not occur, returning to sleep training afterwards is a better solution.

Sleep Training For 10 To 12 Month Old Babies

As stated many times, all babies are different and develop at different times. Many babies are ready for sleep training by their 4th or 5th month but some just don't settle into a sleep pattern until after the 8th month sleep regression. Starting sleep training at this age will be just as effective as doing it earlier and you can generally follow the same steps discussed in the previous chapter. Maintaining consistency will make this much easier. Even if your baby has been resistant to earlier sleep training, keeping a generally constant bed and nap times as well as having a bedtime ritual will make later sleep training more effective.

For older babies, since they have more control of their bodies, the risks of SIDS tend to lower. Adding a special stuffed toy or blanket for your baby to find comfort in, when falling asleep can be beneficial for sleep training at this age. Some methods might consider this a sleep crutch, but as babies age, the comfort object will lose its significance so if it is a crutch it is a short term one and one that doesn't involve the parents which will improve your sleep.

Summary: Sleep At 6 To 12 Months

- Babies at this age tend to move towards sleeping through the night without interruption.
- At 6 months babies will generally sleep 13 to 14 hours a day with 9 to 10 happening at night and the rest in daytime naps
- At one year, babies' nighttime sleep remains constant but their daytime naps will usually decrease in the amount of time by an hour a day.
- A sleep regression usually happens in the 8th to 9th month. In this period, your baby might wake more at night and have shorter or even skipped naps. This period lasts anywhere from a week to 8 weeks.

- Sleep training after the 8th month sleep regression is perfectly acceptable for babies whose sleep schedules have been persistently inconsistent.

Chapter 5: Sleep Training In Other Cultures And Common Baby Sleep Issues

While 'don't compare your baby's development and progress with other babies' has been a bit of a mantra for this book and child rearing in general, but looking at the methods used by other cultures can sometimes provide out of the box thinking. The trend of baby slings in the last 15 to 20 years is an example of a parenting practice that had fallen out of fashion in the western world being reintroduced. Looking at how different cultures handle their babies sleep needs might offer insight that can be used today.

In addition to looking at how other cultures deal with their baby's sleep, this chapter will finish with a look at some of the common sleep issues babies can have, including a couple of the more serious ones. It is important to know the signs and symptoms so that you can consult a pediatrician if needed.

Baby Sleep In Other Cultures

Modern Humans have been around for 40,000 to 50,000 years while the earliest agriculture only dates to about 12,000 years ago. This means that all of the humans living before then were hunter-gatherers. They lived in small groups and foraged for all of their food. Men would generally hunt, often following game for days at a time, while the women of the group would stay closer to their camp and gather what wild food they could find.

Many of them lived in areas with limited resources and would live a nomadic life, moving from place to place often following the migrating game animals, while those lucky enough to live in resource rich areas could live in the same place year round. When it came to babies in hunter-gatherer societies, their mothers would carry them constantly both while she foraged for fruits and nuts and when her tribe moved to a new area.

Outside the mother, these groups of hunter-gatherers often had a collective aspect to their child rearing. The other members of the tribe would often assist mothers when needed. While they were extended groups, they acted more like a close-knit family. In particular, older women in the tribes could act as babysitters as the younger women went about their work. These women were usually mothers themselves, and often grandmothers, so they also taught the younger women the tribe's ways of child rearing.

For nomadic Native Americans, babies in their first year were often carried on a cradleboard. This was a woven or wooden board padded with soft plant fibers like moss, shredded bark, or cattail down. The baby would be strapped onto the board and their mother would then carry their baby with them as they worked or moved with their tribe. These cradleboards often doubled as cribs keeping the baby safe in the night. The constriction of the cradleboard provided the same benefits as the modern swaddling. It also came with the same warnings about hip dysplasia because the baby's legs were often straitened before they were strapped to the cradleboard. Variants of the cradleboard were in use from the Inuit's living above the Arctic Circle to the Tehuelche people of Patagonia.

Help from others in the extended family is a common aspect of ancient childcare that is still in use today in many cultures. Extended families living together in a single household are much more common in Asia, Africa, South America, and parts of Europe. While there are certainly some drawbacks to this situation concerning childcare, the extended family can provide day care for the children of other family members. This comes with the benefit of keeping the baby in a familiar environment that would provide less disruption to the baby's daily nap routine.

Similarly, co-sleeping was common in hunter-gatherer societies as most of them lived in small, often mobile structures where space was at a premium. Co-sleeping is still common in South America, Asia, Africa, and parts of Southern Europe. As stated in chapter 2, there are certainly benefits to this arraignment for both the baby and parents but also disadvantages and warnings. See chapter 2 for more information on co-sleeping.

The Spanish tradition of the siesta or afternoon nap has been losing its prevalence in Spain but in the warmer, southern parts of Europe as well as Latin America, the siesta tradition of returning home for a few hours in the afternoon for a meal and nap offers parents readily scheduled nap that they can share with their babies. Many of the countries were this tradition is still in practice also tend to favor co-sleeping.

Bed times tend to differ in other cultures. The bed times for babies in Europe and Asia are often much later and their babies sleep later into the day. This results in more bonding time with the baby in the evening though this comes at the cost of a few extra hours for the parents themselves after the baby is put to bed. This is also common in areas that favor late dinners. Dinner is often eaten at 9 or 10 o'clock in Latin America, for example so most children's bedtimes happen sometime after that.

Allowing babies to nap outside, though bundled up, is a common practice in Scandinavian countries. This is not just limited to nice sunny days either, but continues even when the outside temperatures are a couple of degrees below freezing. This practice starts as early as 2 weeks old and the outdoor afternoon naps can last as much as three hours. Studies have found that this bracing outdoor naps result in better daytime sleep and longer naps.

While some who practice this in Scandinavia leave their children on their own during these outdoor naps, a more supervised version might be beneficial for other babies in similarly bracing climates. In most climates, sun protection would need to be a part of any baby outdoor napping. Sunburns are often a much more serious condition for babies. Their skin is thinner than adult skin and possesses less protection than adult skin.

Sleep Problems Common In Babies

The vast majority of issues that cause a baby to lose sleep are based on the baby feeling some form of discomfort and are not reasons to seek medical help unless they persist on a continuous basis. The most common of these are hunger, gas, a full diaper, or some sort of injury like a rash. On a more psychological level, separation anxiety can cause some sleeplessness in babies. These minor issues tend to lead to only short-term sleep issues.

Sometimes, however, sleep issues could be part of a larger problem that might require medical help. Some of these include food allergies, acid reflux, sleep apnea, restless leg syndrome, and autism.

Allergies can cause severe gastrointestinal discomfort, which will likely disrupt sleep. Some other symptoms are coughing, diarrhea, rashes, especially around the mouth and a runny nose. Food Protein-Induced Enterocolitis Syndrome (FPIES) is a common allergy that occurs in young infants, symptoms of which often include diarrhea and vomiting 2 to 3 hours after eating. Should this occur on a regular basis, consult a pediatrician.

Acid reflux is a common enough malady for adults but infants can be particularly prone to it. The muscle at the stomach end of the esophagus, the lower esophageal sphincter is not fully developed in young babies. Excessive spitting up after meals as well as squirming at bedtime are possible signs your baby has a reflux issues and you should consult a pediatrician. Keeping your baby upright for a half hour after feeding could also help.

Sleep apnea is a condition that causes short pauses in breathing while sleeping. With a baby, enlarged tonsils are a common cause of this as they enlarge when infected and a baby's immune system is still developing. If your baby is a constant snorer, consult a pediatrician.

Autism is rarely diagnosed in infants and babies but older children who were diagnosed with autism later in life often display a similar set of traits as babies. These include excess squirminess, difficult temperament, impatience, not being cuddly and sleep issues. It is important to note that if your baby exhibits these traits, it doesn't mean they are autistic, but consulting a pediatrician is often warranted.

A fidgety baby at bedtime that just can't settle down might be dealing with restless leg syndrome. This is a movement disorder that causes an overwhelming desire to move their legs, often at bedtime. This leads to both less sleep and a drop in sleep quality. It often runs in families and is more common in women than men are, so mothers with restless leg syndrome whose babies exhibit these signs might have a possible answer.

Appendix: Sources Used

https://www.babysleep.com

https://www.babycenter.com/baby-sleep-basics

https://www.parents.com/baby

https://amotherfarfromhome.com/ultimate-newborn-sleep-schedule-week-by-week/

https://www.parents.com/baby/care/newborn/why-is-routine-important-for-babies/

https://www.parenting.com/article/4-most-important-baby-routines

https://www.parents.com/baby/sleep/basics/understanding-baby-sleep-4-6-months/?slideId=slide_2c36d144-70df-4ef2-bd2b-98aa34d8e8d4#slide_2c36d144-70df-4ef2-bd2b-98aa34d8e8d4

https://www.thebump.com/a/how-to-sleep-train

https://www.babysleepsite.com/sleep-training/baby-toddler-sleep-cultural-differences/

https://www.happiestbaby.com/blogs/blog/first-year-sleep-schedule

https://www.babysleepsite.com/baby-sleep-patterns/sleep-regressions/

https://www.psychologytoday.com/us/blog/singletons/201010/raising-baby-hunter-gatherer-style

https://www.parentingscience.com/infant-sleep-problems.html

http://sleepeducation.org/sleep-disorders-by-category/sleep-breathing-disorders/infant-sleep-apnea/overview-facts

Conclusion

Thank you for making it through to the end of *Baby Sleep Training*. Let's hope it was informative and able to provide you and your baby the chance for a good night sleep.

Just because you have gotten your baby on a sleep schedule that works for both of you, doesn't mean that you can get lax with your baby's sleep hygiene and schedule. A good night's rest is invaluable for your baby's development so keep working to make sure your little one is sleeping soundly and strongly.

Finally, if you found this book useful in any way, a review on Amazon is always appreciated!